100 SLIM FAST DIET RECIPES

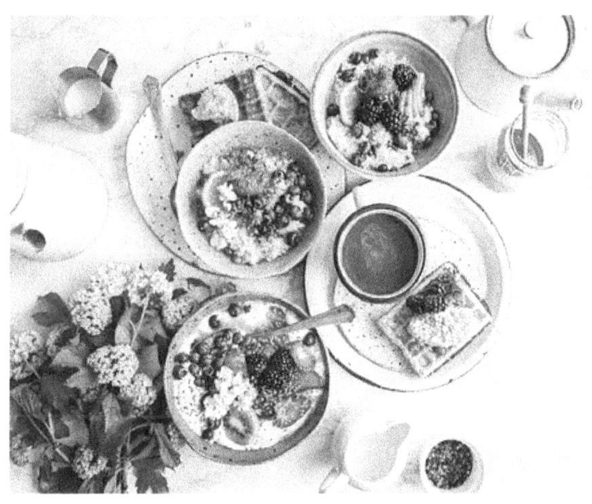

Delicious and Nutritious Recipes to Help You Slim Down Fast

Smart Desty

Copyright © 2023 by [Smart Desty]

This book is a work of nonfiction. While some of the names of people, places, and events have been changed, the author has made every effort to provide accurate information. The author and publisher are not responsible for any omissions or errors that may occur.

TABLE OF CONTENTS

100 SLIM FAST DIET RECIPES

INTRODUCTION

Do you want to lose weight and keep it off? If so, what diet should you follow? The Slim Fast Diet is a popular and effective diet plan that can help you achieve your weight loss goals. Slim Fast Diet Recipes are a great way to get started on this diet plan. With a variety of delicious and healthy recipes, the Slim Fast Diet is a great option for those looking to lose weight and stay healthy.

100 SLIM FAST DIET RECIPES

CHAPTER ONE:

SLIM FAST DIET BASICS

What Is the Slim Fast Diet?

The Slim Fast Diet is a weight loss plan that focuses on reducing your calorie intake while increasing your protein and nutrient intake. This diet plan involves replacing two of your meals with a low-calorie Slim Fast shake or bar and eating one healthy, balanced meal. The Slim Fast Diet is an easy way to reduce your calorie intake and can help you reach your desired weight.

Benefits of the Slim Fast Diet

The Slim Fast Diet provides many benefits to those looking to lose weight. This diet plan is designed to reduce your calorie intake while increasing your protein and nutrient intake, making it an effective way to lose weight. Additionally, the Slim Fast Diet is easy to follow and can be tailored to fit your individual needs.

Slim Fast Diet Recipes are an important part of this diet plan. These recipes provide a variety of healthy and delicious meals that can help you stick to the Slim Fast Diet and reach your weight loss goals. From meals that focus on protein to snacks that are high in fiber, there are many recipes that can help you stay on track.

Breakfast Recipes

Breakfast is an important part of the Slim Fast Diet and there are many delicious and healthy breakfast recipes to choose from. From omelets to smoothies, there are plenty of options for a great start to the day. Some of the most popular breakfast recipes include egg white omelets, Greek yogurt smoothies, and overnight oats.

Lunch Recipes

Lunch is an important part of the Slim Fast Diet and there are many delicious and healthy lunch recipes to choose from. From salads to soups, there are plenty of options for a nutritious and tasty lunch. Some of the most popular lunch recipes include Greek salad, turkey and veggie wrap, and minestrone soup.

Dinner Recipes

Dinner is an important part of the Slim Fast Diet and there are many delicious and healthy dinner recipes to choose from. From stir-fries to burgers, there are plenty of options for a nutritious and tasty dinner. Some of the most popular dinner recipes include teriyaki chicken stir-fry, veggie burgers, and grilled salmon.

Snack Recipes

Snacks are an important part of the Slim Fast Diet and there are many delicious and healthy snack recipes to choose from. From smoothies to trail mix, there are plenty of options for healthy snacks that will help you stay on track. Some of the most popular snack recipes include smoothie bowls, trail mix, and hummus with veggies.

The Slim Fast Diet is a popular and effective diet plan that can help you reach your weight loss goals. Slim Fast Diet Recipes are a great way to get started on this diet plan. With a variety of delicious and healthy recipes, the Slim Fast Diet is a great option for those looking to lose weight and stay healthy. Whether you're looking for breakfast, lunch, dinner, or snack recipes, there are plenty of options to choose from. Choose the Slim Fast Diet today and start on your weight loss journey.

CHAPTER TWO:

HEALTHY SLIM FAST BREAKFAST RECIPES

1. **Overnight Oats with Yogurt and Berries**: Combine ½ cup oats, ½ cup plain yogurt, ½ cup berries, and 2 tablespoons of chia seeds. Refrigerate overnight and enjoy in the morning.

2. **Avocado Toast with Egg**: Toast 2 slices of whole-grain bread. Top with ½ mashed avocado, a sprinkle of salt, and 1 poached or fried egg.

3. **Breakfast Burrito**: Fill a whole-wheat tortilla with scrambled eggs, black beans, and salsa.

4. Smoothie Bowl: Blend ½ cup frozen fruit, ½ cup Greek yogurt, and ¼ cup of milk. Pour into a bowl and top with sliced banana, nuts, and coconut flakes.

5. Egg and Cheese Sandwich: Toast 2 slices of whole-grain bread. Layer with 1 fried egg, 1 slice of cheese, and lettuce.

6. Protein Pancakes: Whisk together 2 eggs, 1 scoop of protein powder, and 1 tablespoon of almond butter. Cook in a non-stick pan over medium heat.

7. Savory Oatmeal: Cook ½ cup of oats in 1 cup of water. Stir in ½ cup of grated cheese, 2 tablespoons of chopped fresh herbs, and a pinch of salt and pepper.

8. **Yogurt Parfait**: Layer ½ cup Greek yogurt, ½ cup granola, and ½ cup of fresh fruit.

9. **Breakfast Quesadilla**: Spread ½ cup grated cheese on a whole-grain tortilla. Top with 1 scrambled egg, diced tomato, and chopped spinach. Fold and cook in a non-stick pan over medium heat.

10. **Breakfast Pizza**: Spread ½ cup tomato sauce on a whole-wheat pita. Top with 1 scrambled egg, grated cheese, and diced bell peppers. Bake at 350°F for 10 minutes.

11. **Veggie Frittata**: Whisk together 8 eggs and a splash of milk. Pour into a pre-heated skillet and top with mushrooms, bell peppers, and spinach. Bake at 350°F for 20 minutes.

12. **Chia Pudding**: Combine 2 tablespoons of chia seeds with ½ cup of coconut milk and ½ cup of plain yogurt. Refrigerate overnight and top with fresh fruit in the morning.

13. **Muffin Tin Omelets**: Whisk together 8 eggs and a splash of milk. Divide the mixture among 6 greased muffin cups. Top with grated cheese, diced bell peppers, and chopped spinach. Bake at 350°F for 20 minutes.

14. **Breakfast Sandwich**: Toast 2 slices of whole-grain bread. Layer with 1 fried egg, 1 slice of cheese, and sliced tomato.

15 **Turkey Bacon and Egg Wraps**: Wrap 2 strips of turkey bacon and 1 fried egg in a whole-wheat tortilla.

16. **Whole-Grain Waffles**: Whisk together 1 cup of whole-grain flour, 2 tablespoons of

baking powder, and 2 eggs. Cook in a waffle iron and top with fresh fruit and a drizzle of maple syrup.

17. **Feta and Spinach Scramble**: Scramble together 4 eggs, ½ cup of feta cheese, and ½ cup of cooked spinach.

18. **Oatmeal with Apples and Cinnamon**: Cook ½ cup of oats in 1 cup of water. Stir in 1 diced apple, 1 teaspoon of cinnamon, and a pinch of salt.

19. **Breakfast Tacos**: Fill a whole-wheat tortilla with 1 scrambled egg, grated cheese, and diced tomatoes.

20. **Banana Peanut Butter Toast**: Toast 2 slices of whole-grain bread. Spread with 2 tablespoons of peanut butter and top with sliced banana.

100 SLIM FAST DIET RECIPES

CHAPTER THREE:
HEALTHY SLIM FAST SNACK RECIPES

1. **Chocolate Covered Peanut Butter Protein Bites**: Combine one cup of creamy peanut butter, one cup of honey, and one cup of vanilla protein powder. Roll into 1-inch balls and dip each one into melted dark chocolate. Refrigerate until hardened.

2. **Avocado Toast with Sunflower Seeds**: Toast two slices of whole grain bread. Spread with mashed avocado and sprinkle with sunflower seeds.

3. **Banana and Almond Butter Roll-Ups**: Spread almond butter on two slices of whole wheat bread. Place a banana in the center and roll up.

4. **Apple Sandwiches with Peanut Butter**: Spread peanut butter on two slices of whole wheat bread. Place thinly sliced apples in the center and close the sandwich.

5. **Greek Yogurt with Fresh Berries**: Top a cup of Greek yogurt with fresh berries and a sprinkle of granola.

6. **Baked Apples with Walnuts and Raisins**: Core one apple and fill the center with raisins and chopped walnuts. Bake for 20 minutes at 350 degrees.

7 **Trail Mix**: Combine ¼ cup of raisins, ¼ cup of almonds, ¼ cup of sunflower seeds, and ¼ cup of dried cranberries.

8. **Hummus and Veggie Sticks**: Serve hummus with fresh vegetables such as carrots, celery, and bell peppers.

9. Frozen Yogurt Bark: Spread plain Greek yogurt on a baking sheet lined with parchment paper. Sprinkle with your favorite nuts and freeze until solid.

10. Protein Smoothies: Blend together a scoop of your favorite protein powder, one banana, ½ cup of almond milk, and a handful of spinach.

11. Whole Wheat Crackers with Cheese and Apples: Top whole wheat crackers with shredded cheese and thinly sliced apples.

12. Peanut Butter and Banana Toast: Spread peanut butter on two slices of whole wheat toast. Top with sliced bananas and a sprinkle of cinnamon.

13. Edamame: Boil edamame in salted water for 3 minutes. Drain and enjoy.

14. Guacamole with Baked Tortilla Chips: Mash one ripe avocado in a bowl. Add a pinch of salt and lime juice. Serve with baked tortilla chips.

15. Celery and Cream Cheese: Spread cream cheese on celery sticks and sprinkle with your favorite herbs.

16. Cucumber Salad: Thinly slice one cucumber and mix with ¼ cup of plain Greek yogurt and a pinch of salt.

17. Popcorn: Pop your own popcorn in a pot and sprinkle with a pinch of salt.

18. Sliced Apples with Almond Butter: Slice one apple and spread each slice with almond butter.

19. Zucchini Chips: Slice one zucchini into thin rounds. Olive oil should be added before baking for 20 minutes at 400 degrees.

20 Overnight Oats: Combine ½ cup of oats, 1 cup of almond milk, 1 tablespoon of chia seeds, and a pinch of cinnamon in a jar. Let sit overnight in the refrigerator.

CHAPTER FOUR:
HEALTHY SLIM FAST LUNCH RECIPES

1. Avocado and Egg Salad Sandwich: Spread a layer of mashed avocado on multigrain bread, top with a boiled egg, salt and pepper, and lettuce.

2. Mediterranean Wrap: Spread hummus on a whole wheat tortilla wrap, add roasted red peppers, feta cheese, olives, and a handful of baby spinach.

3. Veggie and Bean Burrito: Spread a layer of refried beans on a whole wheat tortilla wrap, add grated cheese, diced tomatoes, diced onions, and bell peppers.

4. Turkey and Hummus Sandwich: Spread a layer of hummus on multigrain bread, top with turkey slices, lettuce, and tomato.

5. Greek Salad: Combine chopped cucumbers, tomatoes, feta cheese, olives, and lemon juice.

6. Veggie Quesadilla: Spread a layer of refried beans on a whole wheat tortilla wrap, add grated cheese, diced tomatoes, diced onions, and bell peppers.

7. Hummus and Veggie Pita: Spread a layer of hummus on a whole wheat pita, top with lettuce, diced tomatoes, cucumbers, and feta cheese.

8. Turkey and Avocado Sandwich: Spread a layer of mashed avocado on multigrain bread, top with turkey slices, salt and pepper, and lettuce.

9. Lentil Salad: Combine cooked lentils with feta cheese, diced tomatoes, diced cucumbers, and a light vinaigrette.

10. Spinach and Feta Wrap: Spread a layer of hummus on a whole wheat tortilla wrap, add crumbled feta cheese, baby spinach, and diced tomatoes.

11. Egg Salad Sandwich: Mash boiled eggs with a fork, spread on multigrain bread, add mustard, salt and pepper, and lettuce.

12. Turkey and Cheese Wrap: Spread a layer of mayonnaise on a whole wheat tortilla wrap, top with turkey slices, grated cheese, and lettuce.

13. **Asian Coleslaw**: Combine shredded cabbage, grated carrots, diced green onions, and a light sesame oil-based dressing.

14. **Tuna Salad Sandwich**: Mash canned tuna with a fork, spread on multigrain bread, add diced celery, mayonnaise, and lettuce.

15. **Grilled Veggie Sandwich**: Grill bell peppers, onions, and mushrooms, spread a layer of hummus on multigrain bread, top with the grilled vegetables.

16. **Quinoa Salad**: Combine cooked quinoa with shredded carrots, diced tomatoes, black beans, and a light vinaigrette.

17. **Turkey and Hummus Wrap**: Spread a layer of hummus on a whole wheat tortilla

wrap, top with turkey slices, lettuce, and diced tomatoes.

18. Greek Yogurt and Fruit Parfait: Layer Greek yogurt, diced fruit of your choice, and chopped nuts in a bowl.

19. Caprese Sandwich: Spread a layer of pesto on multigrain bread, top with sliced tomatoes, fresh mozzarella, and fresh basil.

20. Egg, Spinach, and Cheese Wrap: Spread a layer of mayonnaise on a whole wheat tortilla wrap, top with a boiled egg, baby spinach, grated cheese, and diced tomatoes.

35

CHAPTER FIVE:
HEALTHY SLIM FAST DINNER RECIPES

1. **Grilled Chicken with Tomatoes and Mushrooms**: Cook chicken breasts on a hot grill. Top with sliced tomatoes and mushrooms and a sprinkle of garlic and herbs. Serve with a side of steamed broccoli.

2. **Zucchini Fritters**: Shred zucchini and mix with an egg, garlic, and herbs. Heat a non-stick skillet with olive oil and drop tablespoonfuls of the mixture in. Cook until golden brown and serve with a side of Greek yogurt.

3. **Salmon and Spinach Salad**: Cook salmon in a pan and set aside. In a bowl, mix spinach, tomatoes, feta cheese, and a light

vinaigrette dressing. Place the salmon on the salad and sprinkle with herbs.

4. Portobello Burger: Slice a portobello mushroom into thin slices and cook in a pan with olive oil. Serve on a whole-wheat bun with lettuce, tomato, and a light mayonnaise.

5. Baked Tilapia with Asparagus: Place tilapia fillets in a baking dish and top with sliced asparagus spears. Sprinkle with garlic and herbs and bake for 20 minutes. Serve with a side of brown rice.

6. Oven Baked Chicken and Vegetables: Cut up a chicken breast into cubes and place in a baking dish. Top with a variety of vegetables, such as bell peppers, onions, and mushrooms. Drizzle with olive oil and bake for 45 minutes.

7. Broccoli and Cheese Stuffed Peppers: Cut bell peppers in half and remove the seeds. Fill with a mixture of cooked broccoli, grated cheese, and herbs. Bake for 30 minutes or until the peppers are tender.

8. Black Bean and Quinoa Bowl: Cook quinoa according to package instructions. In a separate pan, heat black beans with garlic, onion, and cilantro. Mix the quinoa and black beans together and serve with a side of salsa.

9. Turkey Tacos: Slice turkey and cook in a pan. Place a spoonful of the cooked turkey in a warm tortilla and top with lettuce, tomatoes, cheese, and a light sour cream.

10. Seared Salmon with Dill Sauce: Cook salmon fillets in a skillet and serve with a dill sauce made from Greek yogurt and fresh dill. Serve with roasted potatoes and steamed vegetables.

11. Turkey and Avocado wraps: Cut turkey into strips and cook in a pan with olive oil. Place the turkey in a wrap with lettuce, sliced avocado, and a light mayonnaise.

12. Stuffed Peppers with Quinoa: Cut bell peppers in half and remove the seeds. Fill with a mixture of cooked quinoa, black beans, corn, and herbs. Bake for 30 minutes or until the peppers are tender.

13. Cauliflower Fried Rice: Pulse cauliflower in a food processor until it looks like rice. Heat a skillet with olive oil and add the cauliflower "rice" along with vegetables and herbs. Cook for 10 minutes and serve.

14. Chicken and Broccoli Stir Fry: Heat a skillet with olive oil and add chicken strips. Once the chicken is cooked, add broccoli and stir fry for 3-4 minutes. Serve with a side of brown rice.

15. Tofu and Veggie Curry: Heat a pan with olive oil and add diced tofu. Once the tofu is cooked, add vegetables, such as bell peppers and mushrooms. Add curry powder and simmer for 10 minutes. Serve with quinoa.

16. Lentil Tacos: Cook lentils according to package instructions. Place a spoonful of the cooked lentils in a warm tortilla and top with lettuce, tomatoes, and a light sour cream.

17. Veggie Burrito Bowl: Cook quinoa according to package instructions. In a separate pan, heat black beans with garlic, onion, and cilantro. Mix the quinoa and black beans together and serve in a bowl with vegetables and a light sour cream.

18. Turkey and Zucchini Meatballs: Mix ground turkey with shredded zucchini, garlic, and herbs. Form into small balls and bake for 15 minutes. Serve with a side of steamed vegetables.

19. Baked Eggplant Parmesan: Cut eggplant into thin slices, brush with olive oil, and bake for 15 minutes. Top with marinara sauce and grated cheese and bake for 10 minutes.

20. Grilled Vegetable Platter: Slice a variety of vegetables, such as bell peppers, onions, zucchini, and mushrooms. Grill the vegetables in a hot skillet until they are tender. Serve with a side of hummus.

CHAPTER SIX:
HEALTHY DESSERT RECIPES

1. **Peanut Butter Banana Protein Pudding** – Blend 1 banana, 1/4 cup peanut butter, 1/4 cup plain Greek yogurt, and 1 scoop of protein powder. Serve chilled.

2. **Strawberry Banana Coconut Smoothie** – Blend 1 banana, 1/2 cup strawberries, 1/4 cup shredded coconut, 2 tablespoons Greek yogurt, and 1 scoop of protein powder.

3. **Chocolate Chip Coconut Protein Bars** – Mix 1/4 cup coconut oil, 1/4 cup honey, 1/2 cup almond butter, 1/2 cup coconut flakes, 1/2 cup chocolate chips, and 1 scoop of protein powder. Press into an 8x8 inch pan and freeze.

4. Almond Butter Protein Cups – Mix 1/4 cup almond butter, 1/4 cup honey, 1/4 cup coconut flakes, and 1/2 scoop of protein powder. Press into cupcake liners and freeze.

5. Chocolate Peanut Butter Protein Shake – Blend 1 banana, 1/4 cup peanut butter, 1/2 cup almond milk, 2 tablespoons cocoa powder, and 1 scoop of protein powder.

6. Pumpkin Pie Protein Pudding – Blend 1/2 cup pumpkin puree, 1/4 cup Greek yogurt, 1/4 cup almond milk, 1 teaspoon pumpkin pie spice, and 1 scoop of protein powder.

7. Banana Oatmeal Protein Bars – Mix 1/4 cup honey, 1/4 cup coconut oil, 1 banana, 1/2 cup oats, 1/4 cup almond butter, and 1 scoop of protein powder. Press into an 8x8 inch pan and freeze.

8. Chocolate Coconut Protein Parfait – Layer 1/4 cup Greek yogurt, 1/4 cup shredded coconut, 1/2 banana, 1 tablespoon cocoa powder, and 1 scoop of protein powder.

9. Protein Shake with Peanut Butter – Blend 1 banana, 1/2 cup almond milk, 1 scoop of protein powder, 1/4 cup peanut butter, and 2 teaspoons chocolate powder.

10 Apple Cinnamon Protein Bars – Mix 1/4 cup honey, 1/4 cup coconut oil, 1/2 cup oats, 1/2 cup chopped apples, 1 teaspoon cinnamon, and 1 scoop of protein powder. Press into an 8x8 inch pan and freeze.

11. Vanilla Almond Protein Shake – Blend 1 banana, 1/4 cup almond butter, 1/2 cup almond milk, 1 teaspoon vanilla extract, and 1 scoop of protein powder.

12. Chocolate Coconut Protein Balls – Mix 1/4 cup shredded coconut, 1/4 cup almond butter, 1 tablespoon cocoa powder, 1/4 cup honey, and 1 scoop of protein powder. Roll into balls and freeze.

13. Peanut Butter Cup Protein Parfait – Layer 1/4 cup Greek yogurt, 1/4 cup peanut butter, 1/2 banana, 1 tablespoon cocoa powder, and 1 scoop of protein powder.

14. Apple Pie Protein Shake – Blend 1/2 cup applesauce, 1/4 cup Greek yogurt, 1/4 cup almond milk, 1 teaspoon cinnamon, 1 teaspoon nutmeg, and 1 scoop of protein powder.

15. Peanut Butter Banana Protein Parfait – Layer 1/4 cup Greek yogurt, 1/4 cup peanut butter, 1/2 banana, and 1 scoop of protein powder.

16. Chocolate Coconut Protein Shake – Blend 1 banana, 1/4 cup shredded coconut, 2 tablespoons cocoa powder, 1/2 cup almond milk, and 1 scoop of protein powder.

17. Blueberry Coconut Protein Bars – Mix 1/4 cup coconut oil, 1/4 cup honey, 1/2 cup almond butter, 1/2 cup coconut flakes, 1/2 cup fresh blueberries, and 1 scoop of protein powder. Press into an 8x8 inch pan and freeze.

18. Almond Butter Chocolate Protein Bars – Mix 1/4 cup almond butter, 1/4 cup honey, 1/2 cup chopped almonds, 2 tablespoons cocoa powder, and 1 scoop of protein powder. Press into an 8x8 inch pan and freeze.

19. Chocolate Peanut Butter Protein Balls – Mix 1/4 cup peanut butter, 1/4 cup honey, 2 tablespoons cocoa powder, 1/4 cup oats, and 1 scoop of protein powder. Roll into balls and freeze.

20. Banana Oatmeal Protein Parfait – Layer 1/4 cup Greek yogurt, 1/4 cup oats, 1/2 banana, 1/4 cup almond butter, 1/4 cup chopped walnuts, and 1 scoop of protein powder.

CONCLUSION

The Slim Fast diet is a popular meal replacement diet that has been around for many years. It is a great way to lose weight quickly and safely, while still getting all the nutrients your body needs. It is also an easy way to follow a healthy diet on a budget. The diet consists of replacing two meals a day with a Slim Fast shake or bar, and then eating a healthy, balanced meal or snack for the remaining meal.

The Slim Fast diet has many benefits, such as helping to reduce calorie intake while still providing all the essential nutrients needed for a healthy diet. It also helps to reduce hunger and cravings as well as providing a convenient way to follow a healthy diet.

In addition to the meal replacements, it is important to add healthy snacks and meals to the diet to ensure that all essential nutrients are being consumed. Eating a variety of protein sources (lean meats, fish, eggs, beans, and low-fat dairy products) and fiber-rich fruits, vegetables, and whole grains is important for a healthy diet, as well as drinking plenty of water.

The Slim Fast diet can be a great way to jump-start weight loss and make it easier to stay on track with a healthy diet. There are a variety of Slim Fast diet recipes available online, including smoothies, bars, and shakes, as well as breakfast, lunch, and dinner recipes. All of these recipes can be made with ingredients that are affordable and easy to find.

In conclusion, the Slim Fast diet is a convenient and effective way to lose weight quickly and safely. It can be a great way to jump-start a weight-loss journey and make it easier to stay on track with a healthy diet. The diet consists of replacing two meals a day with a Slim Fast shake or bar, and then eating a healthy, balanced meal or snack for the remaining meal. Additionally, it is important to add healthy snacks and meals to the diet to ensure that all essential nutrients are being consumed. There are a variety of Slim Fast diet recipes available online, making it easy to find recipes that are both tasty and nutritious.